The Heart of Athletic Care: Daily Devotions for Christian Athletic Trainers

Delightful Devotionals

CONTENTS

Introduction — 6

Day 1: The Athletic Trainer's Calling — 9

Day 2: Strength in Compassion — 13

Day 3: Overcoming Challenges — 17

Day 4: The Power of Resilience — 21

Day 5: Rest and Recovery — 25

Day 6: Teamwork and Support — 29

Day 7: Self-Care for Athletic Trainers — 33

Day 8: Encouragement in Scripture — 37

Day 9: Trusting in God's Plan — 41

Day 10: Finding Joy in Service — 45

Day 11: Patience in Adversity — 49

Day 12: A Heart of Gratitude — 53

Day 13: The Healing Power of Prayer — 57

Day 14: Finding Balance — 62

Day 15: Encouraging Others — 67

Day 16: Wisdom and Discernment — 71

Day 17: Building a Legacy — 74

Day 18: The Promises of God — 79

Day 19: Staying Grounded in Faith — 83

Day 20: Celebrating Success — 88

Day 21: Renewed and Empowered — 92

Conclusion — 97

Notes — 99

Introduction

Welcome to "The Heart of Athletic Care - Daily Devotions for Christian Athletic Trainers" This book is specially crafted for those who hold one of the most vital yet often unsung roles in the world of sports – athletic trainers. It is for those who, through their dedication, expertise, and unwavering commitment, contribute to the well-being and success of athletes across the globe.

As an athletic trainer, you stand at the intersection of passion and perseverance, where the desire for excellence in sports meets the challenges of physical health. You are not merely a healthcare provider; you are a vital pillar of support for athletes, helping them overcome injuries, navigate physical demands, and perform at their best. Your work often goes unnoticed, but its impact reverberates on fields, courts, and tracks, where dreams become realities.

Amidst the demands of this profession, it can be easy to forget to care for yourself. The long hours, the emotional rollercoaster of victories and setbacks, and the ongoing pursuit of excellence can be physically and emotionally draining. This devotional is a 21-day devotional journal designed to provide you, the caregiver, with the care and encouragement you need.

Throughout these 21 days, we will explore themes that resonate not only with the world of athletic training but also with your personal and spiritual well-being. The scriptures will be our guide, offering wisdom, hope, and renewal. Practical encouragement and journal questions will accompany these teachings, making the insights relevant and relatable to your life.

So, as we embark on these 21 days together, open your heart, find moments of stillness, and allow yourself to be encouraged, renewed, and empowered. You are not alone; the wisdom, grace, and love of God will accompany you on this path of caregiving and self-discovery.

Day 1: The Athletic Trainer's Calling

Verse of the Day:

"Each of you should use whatever gift you have received to serve others, as faithful stewards of God's grace in its various forms." - 1 Peter 4:10 (NIV)

Reflection:

In the world of athletics, injuries and setbacks are inevitable. However, it is your unwavering commitment and dedication that help athletes overcome these challenges and emerge stronger. You are the guardian of their well-being, supporting them through the highs and lows of their sporting careers.

Athletic trainer, you have been entrusted with a unique and impactful calling. You are not just a healthcare provider; you're a healer, educator, and mentor. Your daily work extends far beyond diagnosing injuries and taping ankles; it's about mending spirits, nurturing dreams, and guiding athletes on their journey to success. You are a faithful steward of the diverse talents and skills you possess, using them to serve others in the realm of sports and physical well-being.

Reflect today on your calling as an athletic trainer. Consider the passion that led you to this profession and the countless lives you've touched along the way. Think about the athletes who have found solace and strength in your care. Your work is not just a job; it's a divine mission.

Encouragement:

As you begin this 21-day journey, let's start with acknowledging the importance of your calling. You are a vital part of the sports world, and your role has a lasting impact. Embrace your mission with renewed purpose and passion, for you are not just an athletic trainer; you are a beacon of hope and healing. Your skills, your knowledge, and your heart make a significant difference in the lives of athletes.

Journal:

1. Reflect on your journey. What initially drew you to this profession, and how has your calling evolved over time?
2. Think about a specific athlete or individual you've had the privilege of serving. How did your role as an athletic trainer impact their physical and emotional well-being? What was the most rewarding aspect of this experience?
3. Consider how your calling as an athletic trainer is a form of stewardship of your skills and knowledge. In what ways can you further develop your abilities to better serve others in the field of sports and physical well-being?

Day 2: Strength in Compassion

Verse of the Day:

"Finally, all of you, be like-minded, be sympathetic, love one another, be compassionate and humble." - 1 Peter 3:8 (NIV)

Reflection:

Compassion is at the heart of what you do as an athletic trainer. It's the unwavering empathy you extend to those in your care, a powerful force that can bring comfort and healing in times of pain and uncertainty. The field of athletics often pushes people to their limits, both physically and mentally. In these moments, your compassion serves as a beacon of light, guiding athletes through their darkest hours.

The Bible tells us stories of compassion, revealing how this virtue has the power to heal, restore, and uplift. The parable of the Good Samaritan, for instance, demonstrates the impact of showing compassion to those in need. In the world of sports, there are countless examples of athletes who have overcome adversity, often with the help of a compassionate trainer by their side.

As you reflect on your role, consider the athletes you've cared for. Think of the moments when a simple act of kindness or a comforting word made all the difference. Your compassion provides the strength that enables athletes to endure pain, recover, and return to the game they love.

Encouragement:

Today, take a moment to appreciate the compassion that flows through your veins as a caregiver. It's not just about physical healing; it's about healing hearts and nurturing the spirit. Your compassion is a precious gift that brings hope and strength to those you serve.

Journal:

1. Reflect on a specific experience where your compassion as an athletic trainer made a significant impact on an athlete's journey. How did your empathy and support help them navigate a challenging situation?

2. Think about the ways you've drawn inspiration from stories of compassion in the Bible or real-life sports scenarios. How have these stories influenced your own approach to your profession?

3. Consider how you can further cultivate and express compassion in your role as an athletic trainer. Are there specific areas in which you can enhance your empathy and care for the athletes under your guidance?

Day 3: Overcoming Challenges

Verse of the Day:

"I can do all this through him who gives me strength." - Philippians 4:13 (NIV)

Reflection:

Being an athletic trainer often means facing a series of challenges and obstacles. It's a profession that demands resilience and unwavering determination. Athletes may encounter injuries, setbacks, and moments of self-doubt. As a trainer, you're there to guide them through these trials and help them overcome adversity.

In the Bible, we find numerous stories of individuals who faced daunting challenges. From David's battle against Goliath to Paul's perseverance through trials, these stories emphasize the importance of relying on God's strength during difficult times. In your role, you can draw inspiration from these scriptures to find the strength to overcome the challenges that come your way.

Your support and encouragement play a vital role in helping athletes push through their limitations and rise above adversity. You are their beacon of hope when they face physical or emotional challenges. Your unwavering faith in their ability to overcome mirrors God's faith in us as we navigate the obstacles of life. Let God be your trainer.

Encouragement:

Today, reflect on the challenges you've encountered as an athletic trainer and how you've helped athletes overcome their own hurdles. Remember the times when your presence, words of encouragement, and unwavering faith have made a difference. You are a source of strength and inspiration for those you serve. Allow God and His Word to be yours.

Journal:

1. Reflect on a specific instance where you helped an athlete overcome a challenging situation. How did your support and unwavering faith make a difference in their journey?
2. Think about a personal challenge you've faced as an athletic trainer. How did your faith and resilience guide you through it?
3. Consider the stories of overcoming challenges in the Bible. Which of these stories resonates with you the most, and how can you draw strength and inspiration from it in your role as an athletic trainer?

Day 4: The Power of Resilience

Verse of the Day:

"Rejoice in hope, be patient in tribulation, be constant in prayer." - Romans 12:12 (ESV)

Reflection:

Resilience is a word often used to describe the ability to bounce back from adversity and to withstand the storms of life. For athletic trainers, resilience is not just a concept but a way of life. It's the unwavering commitment to the athletes under your care, the determination to see them through their toughest challenges, and the resolve to come back stronger after setbacks.

In the Bible, we find stories of resilience that inspire us. Consider the story of Joseph, who faced betrayal, slavery, and imprisonment but emerged as a leader with unwavering faith. Then there's David, who confronted giants and overcame overwhelming odds, all while seeking God's guidance.

In the world of sports, resilience is seen in athletes who bounce back from injuries, teams that rise from the ashes of defeat, and coaches who instill perseverance in their players. It's the spirit that says, "I will not give up."

Encouragement:

As an athletic trainer, your resilience is a guiding light for those you serve. Your ability to stand strong in the face of challenges encourages your athletes to do the same. Embrace the struggles as opportunities to grow, and remember that through it all, you're never alone. Keep rejoicing in hope, be patient in tribulation, and remain steadfast in prayer. Your resilience not only shapes athletes but also molds you into a beacon of strength and inspiration. Stay the course, for you are making a significant impact on and off the field.

Journal:

1. Think about a specific instance where you witnessed an athlete's resilience and determination to overcome adversity. How did their experience inspire you in your role as an athletic trainer?
2. Reflect on a time in your career when you faced a professional challenge or setback. How did your resilience and unwavering faith help you navigate this situation, and what did you learn?
3. Consider the Bible's emphasis on rejoicing in hope, being patient in tribulation, and remaining constant in prayer. How can you integrate these principles into your daily life to further develop your resilience and provide inspiration to those you serve?

Day 5: Rest and Recovery

Verse of the Day:

"Come to me, all you who are weary and burdened, and I will give you rest." - Matthew 11:28 (NIV)

Reflection:

In the world of sports, rest and recovery are essential for athletes to perform at their best. It's during these moments of reprieve that the body heals, rebuilds, and gains strength. As an athletic trainer, the importance of rest and recovery is not only applicable to those you care for but to yourself as well.

You often work tirelessly to ensure the well-being of your athletes, and you know that the demands of your job can be physically and mentally exhausting. Just as athletes require periods of rest to rejuvenate, you too must find moments of solace to recharge your spirits and body.

The Bible reminds us of the rest God provides to those who are weary and burdened. In Him, we find not just physical rest but spiritual rest as well. It's a place where we can cast our cares and find peace.

Encouragement:

Remember that your role is vital, and your work can be strenuous. Don't neglect the importance of taking time for yourself to rest and recover. In those moments of quiet, seek spiritual rest and rejuvenation. Come to the One who understands your weariness, and find the peace that surpasses all understanding. Your ability to care for others is fueled by your own well-being, so take time for rest and reflection. In doing so, you'll not only recharge your spirit but also inspire those around you to embrace the amazing gift of rest and recovery.

Journal:

1. Reflect on a recent moment when you felt physically and emotionally exhausted due to the demands of your role as an athletic trainer. How did you handle this situation, and what did you do to find rest and recovery?

2. Consider the verse from Matthew 11:28, where Jesus invites the weary and burdened to find rest in Him. How can you apply this invitation to your own life and work? What spiritual practices or strategies can help you discover a deeper sense of rest and rejuvenation?

3. Think about the athletes you care for and their attitudes toward rest and recovery. How can you encourage them to prioritize these essential aspects of their training? What lessons from your own journey of rest and recovery can you share with them to inspire their well-being?

Day 6: Teamwork and Support

Verse of the Day:

"Two are better than one because they have a good return for their labor: If either of them falls down, one can help the other up. But pity anyone who falls and has no one to help them up." - Ecclesiastes 4:9-10 (NIV)

Reflection:

Athletic training is a team effort. Whether you're working with professional athletes or students in a school sports program, the importance of teamwork and support cannot be overstated. Just as athletes rely on one another to achieve success, athletic trainers depend on a network of people to provide the best care and support.

The Bible often speaks of the strength found in community and the power of coming together as a team. Ecclesiastes reminds us that two are better than one, and when we have someone to help us up, we can overcome challenges more effectively. In the world of athletic training, this truth is evident daily. The collaborative efforts of trainers, coaches, medical staff, and athletes create an environment in which the team can thrive.

Encouragement:

In the world of athletic training, the power of teamwork and support is indispensable. As you work closely with athletes and fellow professionals, remember that you are part of a team. Embrace this role, knowing that your contribution is invaluable. Seek support when needed, and offer it to others generously. Just as Ecclesiastes reminds us, there is strength in numbers, and in the midst of challenges, it's the support of your team that will lift you up. Lean on your community, and together, you'll continue to make a difference in the lives of athletes and the world of sports.

Journal:

1. Reflect on a memorable experience when the power of teamwork and support became evident in your role. What specific challenges were you able to overcome through the collective efforts of your team, and how did it impact the athletes?

2. Consider the verse from Ecclesiastes 4:9-10. How can you apply the concept of "two are better than one" in your daily work? Are there ways to strengthen your collaborative efforts with other professionals to enhance the support you provide to athletes?

3. Think about the athletes under your care and how they interact with one another. How can you encourage and foster a sense of teamwork and mutual support within the teams or groups you work with? What lessons from your own experience can you share with athletes about the importance of relying on each other for success?

Day 7: Self-Care for Athletic Trainers

Verse of the Day:

"The Lord is my shepherd; I shall not want. He makes me lie down in green pastures. He leads me beside still waters. He restores my soul. He leads me in paths of righteousness for his name's sake." - Psalm 23:1-3 (ESV)

Reflection:

Psalm 23 is a beautiful passage that provides a profound sense of comfort and assurance. In these verses, we find a vivid image of the Lord as our shepherd, guiding us through life's challenges and providing for our needs. The mention of green pastures and still waters reflects the idea of rest and renewal.

As an athletic trainer, you often find yourself in the midst of the fast-paced, demanding sports world, helping athletes navigate their trials and tribulations. These verses encourage you to remember that just as a shepherd cares for the well-being of the flock, God watches over you. He offers you moments of rest, renewal, and soul restoration.

Encouragement:

Let the imagery in Psalm 23 resonate in your heart and mind. The Lord is your Shepherd, and He desires to lead you to places of rest and nourishment, both physically and spiritually. Remember that taking time for self-care and seeking solace is not a sign of weakness but a source of strength. Find comfort in the presence of the Shepherd who guides you, and know that your soul can be refreshed in His care.

Journal:

1. How do you currently incorporate moments of rest and spiritual renewal into your busy life as an athletic trainer?
2. Reflect on times when you've experienced God's guidance and rest in the midst of challenging circumstances. How did it impact your well-being and your ability to support athletes?
3. Consider practical ways to integrate the principles from Psalm 23 into your daily routine to enhance your self-care and spiritual renewal. What steps can you take to allow the Lord to lead you beside still waters and restore your soul?

Day 8: Encouragement in Scripture

Verse of the Day:

"Have I not commanded you? Be strong and courageous. Do not be afraid; do not be discouraged, for the Lord your God will be with you wherever you go." - Joshua 1:9 (NIV)

Reflection:

In the world of athletic training, there are days when you need a powerful dose of encouragement. The Bible is a wellspring of inspiration, offering words of strength, courage, and perseverance. Take a moment to meditate on these verses, allowing them to uplift your spirit and renew your determination.

- *"I can do all things through Christ who strengthens me." - Philippians 4:13 (NIV)*
- *"For God gave us a spirit not of fear but of power and love and self-control." - 2 Timothy 1:7 (ESV)*

- *"But those who hope in the Lord will renew their strength. They will soar on wings like eagles; they will run and not grow weary; they will walk and not be faint." - Isaiah 40:31 (NIV)*
- *"The Lord is my strength and my shield; my heart trusts in him, and he helps me. My heart leaps for joy, and with my song, I praise him." - Psalm 28:7 (NIV)*
- *"He gives strength to the weary and increases the power of the weak." - Isaiah 40:29 (NIV)*

Encouragement:

Draw strength from these words as you face the challenges and demands of your profession. In moments of weariness or uncertainty, remember that God is with you, providing courage and empowerment. Allow the verses to permeate your heart and mind, infusing you with renewed energy and a sense of purpose. You are not alone in your journey as an athletic trainer, and these verses are a reminder of the divine support that surrounds you.

Journal:

1. Which of the provided verses resonates with you the most, and why? How can you apply its message to your role as an athletic trainer when you need encouragement and strength?

2. Reflect on a specific challenging situation or moment in your career when you felt discouraged or apprehensive. How might the verse from Joshua 1:9, "Be strong and courageous," provide

guidance and motivation in such circumstances?

3. In your role as an athletic trainer, you often serve as a source of encouragement for athletes facing adversity. How can these verses on strength and courage inspire you to be an even more impactful source of support and motivation for those you care for?

Day 9: Trusting in God's Plan

Verse of the day:

"Trust in the Lord with all your heart and lean not on your own understanding; in all your ways submit to him, and he will make your paths straight." - Proverbs 3:5-6 (NIV)

Reflection:

In the demanding field of athletic training, where injuries, setbacks, and unexpected challenges are common, it's easy to rely solely on our expertise, experience, and planning. But Proverbs 3:5-6 reminds us that our understanding, though valuable, should not be our sole reliance. Trusting in God's plan means acknowledging that His wisdom surpasses our own, and His path is often filled with lessons, blessings, and divine guidance.

As an athletic trainer, you may face situations that are beyond your control, and it's during these times that trusting in God's plan becomes essential. Choose to surrender your fears, doubts, and anxieties to Him and acknowledge that He has a purpose for every twist and turn in your journey. Even in the face of uncertainty, God's promise to make your paths straight provides the assurance that His guidance is unwavering.

Encouragement:

When challenges arise in your career as an athletic trainer, remember that you're not alone. By trusting in God's plan, you open the door to His divine wisdom and guidance. Let Proverbs 3:5-6 be a source of strength and hope, especially in moments of uncertainty. Embrace His path for you with faith and confidence, knowing that He holds the blueprint for your life's journey.

Journal:

1. Reflect on a time in your career as an athletic trainer when you faced a challenging or uncertain situation. How did you initially approach it? How might trusting in God's plan, as suggested in Proverbs 3:5-6, have influenced your decisions and outlook?

2. Consider the idea of leaning on God's understanding rather than relying solely on your own. How can you incorporate this perspective into your daily work as an athletic trainer, especially when dealing with complex injuries, athlete concerns, or career decisions?

3. Proverbs 3:5-6 encourages us to submit to God in all our ways. How can you actively apply this principle in your professional and personal life? What changes or adjustments can you make to ensure that God's guidance plays a central role in your journey as an athletic trainer?

Day 10: Finding Joy in Service

Verse of the Day:

"Each of you should use whatever gift you have received to serve others, as faithful stewards of God's grace in its various forms." - 1 Peter 4:10 (NIV)

Reflection:

Serving others is not just a responsibility; it's a profound source of joy and fulfillment. As an athletic trainer, you have the privilege of serving athletes and helping them reach their fullest potential. This act of service embodies the love and compassion that Jesus encourages in Matthew 25:40 when He says, "Truly I tell you, whatever you did for one of the least of these brothers and sisters of mine, you did for me."

The joy in service comes from knowing that your skills and dedication can make a significant impact on the lives of others. It's about helping athletes overcome challenges, offering support during their struggles, and being a positive influence in their journey. Joy arises not only from the results you see on the field but also from the transformation that occurs within individuals as they grow, heal, and excel.

Encouragement:

In your role as an athletic trainer, remember that your service is a precious gift. It brings joy not only to those you assist but also to your own life. Find inspiration in the words of Galatians 6:9: "Let us not become weary in doing good, for at the proper time, we will reap a harvest if we do not give up." The joy you discover in service is a testament to the meaningful impact you have on the athletes you support. Even in challenging moments or demanding schedules, find joy in the knowledge that your service is making a difference. Let the love and dedication you pour into your work be a reflection of your faith. By seeing every act of service as an opportunity to share the love of Christ, you can experience profound joy in your role as an athletic trainer.

Journal:

1. Reflect on a specific instance in your career where you found great joy in serving an athlete or team. What made that moment particularly fulfilling, and how did it impact your perspective on your role?

2. How can you ensure that you continue to find joy in service, even during challenging or demanding times in your profession? Are there specific practices or approaches you can adopt to maintain a sense of joy in your work?

3. Consider the idea that your service is a reflection of your faith and an opportunity to share the love of Christ. How can you intentionally integrate your faith into your service, and what difference might this make in the lives of the athletes you serve?

Day 11: Patience in Adversity

Verse of the Day:

"And we boast in the hope of the glory of God. Not only so, but we also glory in our sufferings because we know that suffering produces perseverance; perseverance, character; and character, hope." - Romans 5:2-4 (NIV)

Reflection:

In the world of athletic training, you often face challenging situations and adversity. Athletes may struggle with injuries, setbacks, or moments of self-doubt. During these times, patience becomes a valuable companion. James 1:3-4 reminds us, "The testing of your faith produces perseverance. Let perseverance finish its work so that you may be mature and complete, not lacking anything."

Patience isn't just about waiting; it's about maintaining hope and perseverance when circumstances are tough. It's about trusting that, in time, difficulties can lead to growth and resilience. As an athletic trainer, you play a role in nurturing this patience within athletes as they navigate through adversity.

Encouragement:

When facing adversity, remember the words of Romans 12:12, "Be joyful in hope, patient in affliction, faithful in prayer." Your patience in challenging moments can serve as an inspiration to athletes who may be struggling. Your steadfast presence and commitment to their well-being reflect God's love and care.

Embrace patience as a path to maturity and a testament to your faith. Just as athletes grow stronger through perseverance, your own patience in adversity can lead to personal growth and a deeper sense of purpose in your role as an athletic trainer.

Journal:

1. Reflect on a specific instance in your career where you needed to exercise patience during a challenging situation or adversity. How did patience impact the outcome, and what did you learn?

2. How do you currently nurture patience within the athletes you work with when they face setbacks or difficulties? Are there specific strategies or approaches you use to help them develop perseverance and hope?

3. Consider the idea that adversity can lead to growth and resilience, both for athletes and for yourself. In what ways have you observed these positive outcomes in your journey? How does your faith play a role in your ability to maintain patience and hope in difficult circumstances?

Day 12: A Heart of Gratitude

Verse of the Day:

"Give thanks in all circumstances; for this is God's will for you in Christ Jesus." - 1 Thessalonians 5:18 (NIV)

Reflection:

In the hustle and bustle of athletic training, it's easy to overlook the practice of gratitude. However, maintaining a heart of gratitude is essential for personal well-being and effective service. Gratitude is not limited to the Thanksgiving season; it's a daily habit that can transform your perspective and positively impact those you serve.

In the Bible, we find numerous examples of gratitude. One such instance is when Jesus fed the multitudes with a few loaves and fish. Before multiplying the food, Jesus offered thanks, setting an example of gratitude even in times of scarcity. Similarly, in our daily lives, we can find reasons to be thankful, no matter how challenging our circumstances may be.

Reflect on the moments of gratitude you've experienced in your profession. Perhaps it's the smile of an athlete who has recovered from an injury or the appreciation expressed by a team for your hard work. These moments are reminders of the profound impact you have on the lives of others.

Encouragement:

Embrace gratitude as a way of life. Take time each day to reflect on the blessings in your personal and professional journey. Consider keeping a gratitude journal to record the moments that warm your heart. The habit of gratitude will not only bring joy to your own life but will also inspire those around you.

Journal:

1. Reflect on a recent experience in your career that made you feel particularly grateful. What was the situation, and how did it impact your perspective on your profession and those you serve?
2. How do you currently practice gratitude in your daily life, both personally and professionally? Are there specific routines or rituals you follow to help you maintain a heart of gratitude?
3. Think about the athletes you work with and your colleagues. In what ways can you express your gratitude for their efforts, support, or positive impact on your life? How might sharing your gratitude enhance the relationships and dynamics within your athletic training community?

45

Day 13: The Healing Power of Prayer

Verse of the Day:

"Is anyone among you sick? Let them call the elders of the church to pray over them and anoint them with oil in the name of the Lord. And the prayer offered in faith will make the sick person well; the Lord will raise them up."
- James 5:14-15 (NIV)

Reflection:

In the world of athletic training, healing is a significant aspect of your role. When athletes face injuries or setbacks, they look to you for guidance and support in their journey to recovery. In these moments, prayer can be a powerful tool for healing and strength.

The Bible contains stories of miraculous healings through prayer. In James 5:14-15, we are encouraged to call upon the elders of the church for prayer and anointing when someone is sick. This passage reminds us of the profound healing power of faith-filled prayer. It is a reminder that when we pray with trust and faith, God listens and can bring about healing in both body and spirit.

As an athletic trainer, you may witness injuries and challenges that require more than physical care. Your athletes may also need emotional and spiritual support on their path to recovery. Prayer can offer peace, encouragement, and a sense of God's presence during difficult times. It can be a source of strength not only for the athletes you serve but also for you in your role as a caregiver.

Encouragement:

Today, take a moment to reflect on the healing power of prayer. Consider incorporating prayer into your daily routine for both yourself and the athletes under your care. Recognize that prayer is not just a habit but a lifeline to divine strength and guidance. In times of adversity and injury, remember the words of James 5:14-15 and the promise of healing through faith-filled prayer. Your prayers can bring comfort and healing to those you serve, fostering both physical and spiritual well-being.

Journal

1. Reflect on a specific moment in your athletic training career when you witnessed the impact of prayer on an athlete's healing or recovery. How did this experience influence your perspective on the role of faith and prayer in the healing process?

2. How do you currently integrate prayer or spiritual support into your approach to helping athletes heal and recover from injuries or setbacks? Are there specific practices or rituals that you find effective in providing spiritual care in your profession?

3. In James 5:14-15, we see the importance of community and faith when seeking healing through prayer. How can you encourage and support athletes to engage in faith-filled prayer for their well-being and recovery? Are there ways to create a supportive and spiritually nurturing environment within your athletic training community?

49

Day 14: Finding Balance

Verse of the Day:

"But I have calmed and quieted myself, I am like a weaned child with its mother; like a weaned child, I am content." - Psalm 131:2 (NIV)

Reflection:

Balancing the demands of your profession as an athletic trainer with your personal life can be a significant challenge. The daily responsibilities and unexpected demands can sometimes tip the scales, leaving you feeling overwhelmed. It's essential to remember that finding balance is not just about managing your time but also about seeking contentment in all circumstances.

The verse from Psalm 131:2 paints a beautiful picture of contentment. It likens the psalmist's state of mind to that of a weaned child with its mother—calm, quiet, and content. This verse reminds us of the need for a peaceful and content heart amidst the busyness of life.

As you navigate your career and personal life, it's crucial to find moments of stillness and contentment. Seek God's presence in the midst of your busy schedule, knowing that He offers a sense of peace that transcends circumstances. Balancing your responsibilities requires intentionality and recognizing that true balance is a reflection of the inner peace you find in God's presence.

Encouragement:

Today, take a moment to reflect on the concept of balance in your life. Consider the areas where you may need to find more balance, whether it's in managing your time or seeking contentment amidst life's challenges. Embrace the wisdom of Psalm 131:2 and aim for a heart that is calm and content, regardless of the demands on your schedule. God offers you the gift of inner peace and contentment as you navigate the complexities of your profession and personal life. Trust in Him, and seek balance through His presence.

Journal:

1. Reflect on the moments in your career as an athletic trainer when you felt most balanced and content. What factors contributed to this sense of balance, and how did it impact your overall well-being and effectiveness in your role?

2. Are there specific practices or routines you currently employ to seek moments of stillness and contentment in the midst of your busy schedule? How do these practices help you maintain

balance, and are there new strategies you'd like to explore to enhance your sense of inner peace?

3. How can you integrate the wisdom from Psalm 131:2 into your daily life and profession as an athletic trainer? What steps can you take to approach your responsibilities with a calm and content heart, seeking a sense of balance regardless of external demands?

Day 15: Encouraging Others

Verse of the Day:

"So encourage each other and build each other up, just as you are already doing." - 1 Thessalonians 5:11 (NLT)

Reflection:

As an athletic trainer, you possess a unique ability to encourage and uplift those you serve. Your profession offers opportunities to be a source of motivation, support, and inspiration for athletes and coworkers alike. In doing so, you exemplify the spirit of 1 Thessalonians 5:11 by encouraging one another and building each other up.

Encouragement, in the context of your work, extends beyond the physical aspects of training. It involves offering a word of support when an athlete faces a challenging situation, providing guidance during recovery, or simply being a positive presence. Encouragement is a powerful tool for fostering a spirit of determination and hope.

Consider how you can uplift others today, whether it's through words of affirmation, acts of kindness, or unwavering support. In the world of athletics, your role as an encourager can make a significant impact on the well-being and performance of those under your care.

Encouragement:

Reflect on the opportunities you have had to encourage others throughout your career as an athletic trainer. Think about how your words and actions have made a difference in the lives of athletes and colleagues. Today, take a moment to intentionally encourage someone you interact with, whether it's an athlete, a co-worker, or a friend. Your role as an encourager can have a profound effect, not only on their journey but also on your own sense of fulfillment in your profession. As you build up and support others, you, too, will find encouragement in the process.

Journal:

1. Think of a specific moment in your career as an athletic trainer when you provided encouragement and support to an athlete or colleague. Describe that situation and reflect on the impact your words or actions had on the individual. How did it make you feel to be an encourager in that moment?

2. Consider the athletes or individuals you currently work with. How can you proactively incorporate the principles of 1 Thessalonians 5:11 into your daily interactions with them? What steps can you take to become an even more effective source of encouragement in your professional role?

3. Reflect on a time when someone encouraged you during a challenging moment in your career. How did that encouragement affect your outlook and performance? What qualities or words of encouragement were particularly meaningful to you? How can you replicate these experiences for others in your care?

Day 16: Wisdom and Discernment

Verse of the Day:

"If any of you lacks wisdom, you should ask God, who gives generously to all without finding fault, and it will be given to you." - James 1:5 (NIV)

Reflection:

In the realm of athletic training, making decisions is a daily occurrence. Whether it's determining the best rehabilitation plan for an injured athlete or choosing the most effective training methods, wisdom and discernment are invaluable. James 1:5 reminds us that when we lack wisdom, we can turn to God in prayer, and He will generously provide it.

The decisions you make as an athletic trainer can profoundly impact an athlete's well-being and performance. Your ability to discern the most suitable course of action is a critical aspect of your role. Seeking wisdom not only from your professional knowledge but also from a spiritual perspective can enhance your decision-making process.

Consider how you can incorporate prayer and seeking divine guidance when faced with important choices in your profession. Trust that God's wisdom will help you navigate the complexities of your role and contribute to the well-being of the athletes you serve.

Encouragement:

Today, reflect on a decision you've made in your profession that had a meaningful impact on an athlete's journey. Consider how seeking wisdom and discernment played a role in that decision. As you move forward in your career, remember that you have the opportunity to seek divine guidance in each choice you make. Embrace James 1:5 as a reminder that wisdom is accessible through prayer and faith. Trust that God's wisdom will guide you in making choices that benefit the athletes under your care.

Journal:

1. Think of a specific decision you made as an athletic trainer that required wisdom and discernment. How did you arrive at that decision? Did you seek divine guidance through prayer or reflection? What was the outcome, and what lessons did you learn from this experience?

2. Reflect on a time when you encountered a particularly challenging or complex situation in your role. Did you turn to prayer or seek wisdom from a spiritual perspective to help you make the right decision? How did the presence of divine guidance impact your approach to resolving the issue?

3. In your daily work, consider how you can incorporate the principles of James 1:5 into your decision-making process more regularly. Are there specific areas where you feel the need for greater wisdom and discernment? What steps can you take to make prayer and seeking divine guidance a consistent practice in your career as an athletic trainer?

Day 17: Building a Legacy

Verse of the Day:

"A good name is more desirable than great riches; to be esteemed is better than silver or gold." - Proverbs 22:1 (NIV)

Reflection:

In the world of athletic training, the impact you make on athletes and fellow professionals extends beyond the field or the training room. You are, in essence, building a legacy. Proverbs 22:1 reminds us that a good name, characterized by integrity, respect, and compassion, is more valuable than material wealth.

Your legacy is not defined solely by your accomplishments but by the positive influence you have on the lives of those you encounter. As an athletic trainer, your actions and attitudes can inspire and empower others, leaving a lasting imprint on their journeys.

Consider the kind of legacy you want to build. How do you want to be remembered by the athletes you've supported and the people you've worked with? Reflect on the values and principles that guide your professional life and ensure that they contribute to the legacy you wish to leave.

Encouragement:

Today, take a moment to think about the athletes and individuals you've had the privilege to interact with throughout your career. Consider the positive impact you've had on their lives, whether through your expertise, encouragement, or care. In your role as an athletic trainer, you have the opportunity to build a legacy of compassion, dedication, and excellence. Embrace this opportunity to leave a mark that extends far beyond your professional achievements.

Journal:

1. Reflect on your career as an athletic trainer and the individuals you have worked with. What values or qualities do you hope to be remembered for in your professional legacy? How have you already embodied these qualities, and what steps can you take to further strengthen this legacy?

2. Think of an athlete or colleague you have inspired or positively influenced in your role. What specific actions or attitudes of yours contributed to this impact? How do you envision the ripple effect of this influence in their life and the lives of others?

3. Consider the concept of a "good name" mentioned in Proverbs 22:1. How does the idea of having a good name relate to your role as an athletic trainer and the legacy you are building? What areas of your professional life can benefit from emphasizing integrity, respect, and compassion, as highlighted in the verse?

64

Day 18: The Promises of God

Verse of the Day:

"For I know the plans I have for you, declares the Lord, plans for welfare and not for evil, to give you a future and a hope." - Jeremiah 29:11 (ESV)

Reflection:

God's promises are a source of unwavering hope and assurance in the midst of life's challenges and uncertainties. Jeremiah 29:11 reminds us that God's plans for us are rooted in hope and a promising future.

As an athletic trainer, you may face unexpected hurdles and situations that test your resolve. It's during these times that holding onto the promises of God can provide the strength and faith to persevere. His promises are a testament to His unwavering love and commitment to those who trust in Him.

Take time to meditate on the promises of God, reflecting on the assurance they offer. His promises include guidance, strength, healing, and grace, which are all essential components of your journey as an athletic trainer.

Encouragement:

Carry with you the promises of God as you navigate the challenges and triumphs of your profession. In times of uncertainty or doubt, let His promises be a wellspring of hope, reminding you that you are never alone in your endeavors. Place your trust in His unchanging Word and find the strength and assurance needed to continue your dedicated service as an athletic trainer.

Journal:

1. Reflect on a specific situation in your career as an athletic trainer when you faced challenges or uncertainties. How did trusting in God's promises, like Jeremiah 29:11, provide you with hope and resilience during that time? What were the outcomes of holding onto these promises?

2. Jeremiah 29:11 speaks of God's plans for welfare and a hopeful future. In your role as an athletic trainer, how do you see God's plans manifested in your work? Can you identify moments where you've been part of a plan that brought about welfare and hope for the athletes you've cared for?

3. Take time to list some of God's promises that resonate with you as an athletic trainer. How do these promises influence your approach to your role and your interactions with athletes and colleagues? How can you continue to lean on these promises in your profession to maintain a sense of hope and assurance?

Day 19: Staying Grounded in Faith

Verse of the Day:

"Because of the Lord's great love, we are not consumed, for his compassions never fail. They are new every morning; great is your faithfulness." - Lamentations 3:22-23 (NIV)

Reflection:

In the ever-evolving world of athletic training, the verse from Lamentations 3:22-23 serves as a source of comfort and hope. It reminds us of the Lord's great love and faithfulness, which are steadfast and renewed daily.

As an athletic trainer, you may face daily challenges and uncertainties. There will be moments of triumph and moments of frustration. Yet, in all these experiences, you can find peace in the knowledge that the Lord's love and compassion never waver. His faithfulness is a constant presence in your life.

This verse highlights the idea that each day is a new opportunity. You can begin each morning with a fresh outlook, knowing that the Lord's faithfulness will carry you through. In the midst of your demanding profession, take a moment to appreciate the unwavering love and compassion of your Creator, which can sustain you through the challenges and triumphs of each day.

Encouragement:

Amidst the rigors of your role as an athletic trainer, remember that you are not alone. The faithfulness and love of the Lord are like a wellspring of strength, renewing each day. Take a moment each morning to reflect on this enduring truth. Approach your profession with the understanding that, regardless of the challenges you may face, the Lord's compassion is unending, and His love is your unwavering support. Let this awareness bring you peace and fortitude, knowing that you are held in His faithful embrace.

Journal:

1. Reflect on a specific day in your career as an athletic trainer when you faced unexpected challenges or difficulties. How did the knowledge of the Lord's unwavering love and faithfulness, as mentioned in Lamentations 3:22-23, help you stay grounded and resilient in those moments?

2. Think about how you can apply the concept of "new every morning" from this verse to your daily routine as an athletic trainer. What practices or mindset shifts can you incorporate to

ensure you approach each day with a fresh outlook, aware of God's renewing compassion?

3. Consider your relationship with faith and spirituality in your profession. How does your faith impact your interactions with athletes, colleagues, and the challenges you face as an athletic trainer? In what ways can you further embrace God's faithfulness and compassion as a guiding force in your work?

Day 20: Celebrating Success

Verse of the Day:

"May the God of hope fill you with all joy and peace as you trust in him so that you may overflow with hope by the power of the Holy Spirit." - Romans 15:13 (NIV)

Reflection:

In the world of athletic training, celebrating success can sometimes be overshadowed by the continuous drive for improvement. However, Romans 15:13 reminds us that the God of hope desires to fill us with joy and peace as we trust in Him. This includes moments of celebration.

As an athletic trainer, success may come in various forms, from helping an injured athlete recover to achieving personal and professional goals. It's important to recognize and celebrate these moments. Doing so not only acknowledges your hard work but also allows you to experience the joy and peace that God's hope offers.

The verse from Romans highlights the overflow of hope by the power of the Holy Spirit. This overflow can be seen as the abundance of joy and celebration that comes from recognizing and appreciating your achievements. Celebrating success is a way of embracing hope and experiencing God's joy in your profession.

Encouragement:

Embrace the moments of success in your journey as an athletic trainer. Celebrate the milestones, both big and small, as they come. Rejoice in the progress of those you support in their athletic endeavors. These celebrations are not just for you but also a testament to the hope and joy found in your faith. By acknowledging your achievements, you are living out the hope-filled message of Romans 15:13, allowing the power of the Holy Spirit to fill you with joy and peace.

Journal:

1. Reflect on a recent success or achievement in your career. How did you celebrate this moment, and what feelings of joy and peace did it bring? How did your faith play a role in this celebration?

2. Consider the athletes you've worked with and their achievements. How have you celebrated their successes, and what impact did this have on their motivation and well-being? How might you incorporate more celebrations of their accomplishments into your coaching approach?

3. Explore the concept of hope and its connection to celebration. How does celebrating success not only bring joy and peace to your life but also align with the hope-filled message of Romans 15:13? In what ways can you continue to embrace hope?

Day 21: Renewed and Empowered

Verse of the Day:

"But those who hope in the Lord will renew their strength. They will soar on wings like eagles; they will run and not grow weary; they will walk and not be faint." - Isaiah 40:31 (NIV)

Reflection:

As we conclude this 21-day journey, let the words of Isaiah 40:31 be a source of inspiration. Just as athletes renew their strength and endurance, those who hope in the Lord find a similar renewal. This renewal brings the promise of soaring like eagles, running without growing weary, and walking without growing faint.

Throughout these devotionals, we've explored the challenges and joys of being an athletic trainer and the role your faith plays in your profession. Your work involves caring for the physical well-being of athletes, but it's also a spiritual journey, an opportunity to renew your strength daily.

Take a moment to reflect on the lessons and insights you've gained during this journey. Consider how you've grown in your faith and profession. Know that you have been equipped to continue your calling with the strength of an eagle, running the race set before you without growing weary.

Encouragement:

As you move forward in your role as an athletic trainer, may the promises of Isaiah 40:31 continue to guide you. Renew your hope in the Lord daily. Find inspiration in the strength that only God can provide. Know that, just like the athletes you support, you too can soar to new heights and find endurance to run the race. Your spiritual journey is ongoing, and your faith will empower you in all that you do. Continue to be a beacon of hope and care to the athletes you serve, knowing that your source of strength is the Lord.

Journal:

1. Reflect on the insights and lessons you've gained throughout this 21-day journey. How has your faith been impacted, and in what ways have you grown in your role as an athletic trainer? Are there specific devotionals or verses that have had a profound influence on you?

2. Isaiah 40:31 speaks of finding renewal in hope and strength. How will you actively incorporate the promise of this verse into your daily life and work as an athletic trainer? What strategies or practices can you adopt to ensure that you consistently renew

your strength in the Lord?

3. As you look ahead in your career, how do you envision applying the lessons from this journey to your role as an athletic trainer? How will the combination of faith and profession continue to empower and inspire you, and what positive changes do you anticipate for yourself and the athletes you serve?

Conclusion

Congratulations on completing this 21-day devotional journey designed to encourage and uplift you in your unique profession. We hope this series has served as a source of inspiration and spiritual growth, reminding you of the vital role you play in the lives of athletes and your community.

As you continue your essential work, remember that you are not alone. God's presence is with you, providing strength, wisdom, and compassion. Embrace each day with a spirit of gratitude and a heart filled with the joy of serving others.

We extend our heartfelt gratitude to you for your dedication and commitment to the well-being of athletes. Your profession often goes unsung, but your impact is immeasurable. We encourage you to find moments of rest, reflection, and prayer amidst the demands of your work. Continue seeking inspiration from the Word of God and the support of your faith community.

May this devotional journey serve as a reminder that, as an athletic trainer, you are not just a healer of bodies but a source of hope, encouragement, and inspiration to those you serve. You make a lasting difference in the lives of athletes, and your faith in God's grace empowers you to meet each challenge with strength and resilience.

Thank you for your dedication, and may your journey be filled with purpose, faith, and an enduring spirit of service.

With warmest wishes and gratitude,

Delightful Devotionals